Flexitarian Diet

A Beginner's Step-by-Step Guide with Recipes

Table of Contents

Disclaimer

By reading this disclaimer, you are accepting the terms of the disclaimer in full. If you disagree with this disclaimer, please do not read the book. The content in this book is provided for informational and educational purposes only.

None of the information in this book should be accepted as independent medical or other professional advice.
The information in the books has been compiled from various sources that are deemed reliable. It has been analyzed and summarized to the best of the Author's ability, knowledge, and belief. However, the Author cannot guarantee the accuracy and thus should not be held liable for any errors.

You acknowledge and agree that the Author of this book will not be held liable for any damages, costs, expenses, resulting from the application of the information in this book, whether directly or indirectly. You acknowledge and agree that you assume all risk and responsibility for any action you undertake in response to the information in this book.

You acknowledge and agree that by continuing to read this book, you will (where applicable, appropriate, or necessary) consult a qualified medical professional on this information. The information in this book is not intended to be any sort of medical advice and should not be used in lieu of any medical advice by a licensed and qualified medical professional. Always seek the advice of your physician or another qualified health provider with any issues or questions you might have regarding any sort of medical condition. Do not ever disregard any qualified professional medical advice or delay seeking that advice because of anything you have read in this book.

Introduction

I want to thank you and congratulate you for getting this book.

In recent years, several new diet ideas have emerged, promising quick and easy meal regimens that can burn fat layers in a few weeks. These include the keto diet and intermittent fasting. But if you look closely, these diets actually require a rather strict eating regimen that can take away the fun out of food.

Food is meant to be enjoyed in all its forms, shapes, sizes, texture and taste. The key to enjoying nutritious and tasty meals without the rigid restrictions of the regular diet plan is flexibility – and that is what flexitarian diet is all about.
The term flexitarian comes from the words *flexible + vegetarian* referring to a method of eating that can minimize meat and fat intake without completely removing meat from your diet. A flexitarian diet is ideal for someone who wants to be more of a vegetarian than a carnivore but can't exactly part from the succulent meat dishes. Being a flexitarian offers immense benefits and advantages that you will appreciate.

You will surely gain a fit and shapely body if you obediently stick to the flexitarian diet rules, which are not difficult to follow at all. You may need to create some adjustments in your lifestyle and habits, and this book will guide you from day one of your transition phase.

In order to guide you properly, this book will teach you:

- What flexitarian diet is.
- The dvocacies behind the flexitarian diet.
- The foremost things that you need to do in order to embrace flexitarianism with ease.
- The additional food groups that the diet includes.

- Two options that you can choose from if you follow a flexitarian diet.
- How to do the different recipes that are included and use them to plan your meal.
- Other important things about flexitarian diet.

The flexitarian diet is so flexible that you may never feel like following a certain type of diet at all. The delicious and tempting recipes that are included in this book are enticing and appetizing enough for the whole family to enjoy.

You will gain better health and body in a matter of time, and the best part is you can do the same with the whole family. They won't even notice that they are eating a flexitarian meal, unless you explicitly tell them.

Chapter 1: What is the Flexitarian Diet?

A flexitarian diet consists of plant and animal protein, although it should revolve around plant component more than meat from animals. It offers great flexibility and you won't find it troublesome to follow the diet. In simpler terms, the flexitarian diet allows you to live a vegetarian lifestyle without the need to follow the strictly-plant-food-sources-only rule.

There are flexitarians (people who follow the flexitarian diet) who prefer to have an all-meat diet once a month or on rare occasions, meat-free meal once a week, or meat-free meal for a week. The main idea is that you need to eat more vegetables than meat. Another point that has to be made about flexitarian diet is that it is much more than just about cutting down on meat, and is also about avoiding processed food.

The popularity of flexitarian diet continues to rise. The word 'flexitarian' was first used as early as 2003 and has since then gained its own following. The term was officially added to the Oxford English Dictionary in 2014 as increasingly more and more consumers are starting to abstain from eating pork on a regular basis.

Benefits of being a Flexitarian

First of all, here are a few facts about flexitarians: flexitarians actually weigh less (up to 15 percent less) compared to meat-eaters and are less prone to heart diseases, diabetes, and cancer. Furthermore, people who live on plant-based diets are also expected to live 3.6 years longer compared to others.

People who find it hard to be a vegetarian but still want to get the full advantage of vegetarianism can benefit a lot from following a flexitarian diet. To give you an idea and some incentive to inspire you to begin a flexitarian diet, here are some of its benefits:

Weight loss – studies have revealed that people following a high-vegetable intake diet have body mass indexes (BMIs) that fall within the normal range. When you closely follow flexitarian rules, you can benefit from reduced body fat due to calorie counting. In addition, weight loss is further facilitated with a diet that is low in calories and high in fiber – something that flexitarian diets are known for.

Increased life expectancy – compared to meat-eaters, studies found out that people who eat more fruits, vegetables, nuts and grans have lower risks of contracting cardiovascular diseases and cancer. The flexitarian diet allows for higher intakes of food rich in antioxidants, vitamins, fiber, minerals, and phytochemicals or plant proteins.

Improved metabolism – with fibrous fruits and vegetables integral in the flexitarian diet, your metabolism can never go wrong. There is also emerging evidence that semi-vegetarian diets (SVD) can treat bowel diseases such as Crohn's disease among other inflammatory bowel disorders.

Lower blood sugar – studies are also increasingly pointing out the role that semi-vegetarian diets play in lowering blood glucose levels especially for people living with diabetes. In addition to being an excellent maintenance habit, the flexitarian diet also decreases the risk of acquiring type 2 diabetes.

Overall, flexitarians tend to experience the same benefits that vegetarians and vegans get – from higher life expectancies to lower body weights. But the edge you get from a flexitarian diet lies in the occasional meat intake which remains a necessary source of protein for the human body.

How It Works

In many ways, while the flexitarian diet prides itself for not having excessive diet restrictions, it still follows a scientific approach. The flexitarian diet is meant NOT for people to follow strictly, but as a guide for them to enjoy the benefits of a vegetarian lifestyle with occasional meat and fish intake. This is how it works:

1. In a day, you need to consume a total of 1,500 calories with the following breakdown:
300 calories for breakfast
150 calories for morning snack
400 calories for lunch
150 calories for afternoon snack
500 calories for dinner

If you want to lose weight, you need to strictly follow the calorie intake distribution. It is important to eat your meals on time, but you can adjust the time for your snacks. You can even choose to take your snacks at once (for a total of 300 calories) during a particular time of day when you need to do a tedious task, which requires extra boost of energy. Nevertheless, an increasing number of flexitarians who are not interested in losing weight refrain from calorie counting but still adhere to the 26-ounce rule of meat consumption per week.

2. If you don't want to bother with counting your calories (although it is the best option), you can just limit your consumption of meat to 26 ounces per week and that means you need to eat mostly plant-based foods. The meat part of the diet includes the usual pork and beef plus fish and poultry.

It is important to remember that you should not go beyond the set limit. After all, there are limits to flexibility if you are to consider yourself a flexitarian at all. You can decide for the amount of meat that you need to eat everyday, but keep in mind not to go beyond 26 ounces of meat per week. You can reduce your meat consumption if you want.

3. Meat has always been a part of our daily diet (unless you were trained to eat only vegetables at a young age) and no one can deny that it is too difficult to part from it. Meat is considered one of the most important sources of protein, fat and micronutrients. It is even considered a staple food in most, if not all parts of the globe. But aside from meat, you need to add these food groups when you decide to be a flexitarian:

Vegetables and fruits
Meat alternatives (eggs, tofu, beans, peas, nuts, and other similar foods)
Dairy
Whole grains
Spices and other flavor enhancers

4. Add physical activities in your daily routine to gain additional benefits. You can do simple exercises, jog, walk, Zumba, skipping, swim, play tennis, or anything that can make you sweat. You need to avoid sitting or lying down for a long time. You can also do simple exercises while sitting. Making a point to sweat at least once a day with an intense physical activity is crucial if your goal is to lose weight using a flexitarian diet.

Eating Options

A flexitarian diet is indeed flexible. It is up to you whether to follow the caloric distribution or take the 26 ounces of meat consumption per week into account. You need to do only one. However, it is best to distribute your calorie intake if there's a need for you to lose weight. You can choose from the following options:

1. Every day – eat vegetables with right amount of meat (maximum of 3.7 ounces of meat per day in order to meet the 26-ounce limit).
2. Every Monday – go meat-free. Going for Meatless Mondays is a good habit to form especially when you're just starting with a flexitarian lifestyle. Try this with your friends and family and make sure not to break it for the first twenty-one (21) days in order to turn it into a regular eating habit.
3. Once a week – eat vegetables with a bigger meat portion. Even on your "cheat days," it is vital to integrate vegetables into your meals. There are numerous ways to make vegetables jive effortlessly with bigger meat portions.
4. On rare occasions or once a month – eat a meat-only meal. It's important to keep in mind that this practice should only be done on an occasional basis. Once a month is the recommended period as you will also need the high-protein meal to replenish your protein deposits.

Since it's a flexible diet, it is easy to create a meal plan. You can even incorporate all the eating options in your plan. This book has plenty of recipes that you can mix and match so you can come up with a delicious and healthy meal each time.

Now, transitioning in a completely flexitarian lifestyle can still be a challenge. Various adjustments not just on dietary habits are needed in order to fully transition which is why most flexitarian experts recommend a 'transition period' that paces your dietary track and gears your body for a diet of mostly plant-based food. The transition periods are as follows:

Beginner Phase – 2 meatless days per week (26 oz. of either meat or poultry each week)
Advanced Phase – 3-4 meatless days per week (18 oz. of meat or poultry each week)
Expert – 5 meatless days per week (9 oz. of meat or poultry per week)
If you notice, the phases are divided based on the gradual decrease of meat consumption per week. While the beginner phase of 26 ounces of meat per week works for most people, some advanced and expert flexitarian individuals tend to cut back more on meat and sometimes even fully transition to becoming a pure vegetarian.
Of course, there's no pressure to become a full-fledged vegetarian, but it is important to know that committing to a flexitarian diet is also a means of transitioning into a complete vegetarian.
In many ways, the flexitarian diet is not about reducing meat options for you and your family, but more about adding new meatless dishes for you to enjoy. A flexitarian diet does not necessarily mean you get to eat tofu and salad all day. The core principle behind flexitarianism is actually to provide people with more meatless alternatives and choices so they better understand the food they eat and how excessive meat consumption actually impacts on our health, animal welfare, and the environment as a whole.

Chapter 2: An Environment-Friendly, Sustainable Diet

Flexitarianism is on the rise and has become the popular choice for many citizens including countries like the United Kingdom. According to a recent survey, weekly meat and dairy consumption in the UK have dropped from 1160g per individual in the 1980s to 989g in 2017. This drastic cut in meat and dairy consumption could have been caused by a number of factors including the increasing prices of meat, perceived health benefits of lower meat diets and food scares.

But with the decrease in meat consumption come the rise of sustainable eating habits such as flexitarianism. While veganism and vegetarianism (which include pescatarianism) are widely accepted eating habits, pioneers of the flexitarian diet thought that sustainable eating habits could be more popularly associated with its environmentally sound and sustainable principles if it allowed for a little bit more flexibility – hence, the flexible vegetarian.

The advocacy behind flexitarianism is simple but speaks volumes on the need to change individual lifestyles and community consumption patterns. These are some of the few examples:

Animal welfare – a major consumer base of the flexitarian diet are animal welfare activists and supporters that seek to cut back on meat consumption. Furthermore, these groups wish to end animal cruelty which is something totally unavoidable when we talk about how most meat products are produced today. By cutting down on meat consumption and transitioning to a mainly plant-based diet, the demand for meat (and therefore the amount of animal cruelty practiced) lessens.

Climate change – one of the biggest contributors of greenhouse gas emissions is livestock production which accounts for 14.5 percent of global GHG emissions according to FAO. These GHG emissions come from the demand for livestock feed. For example, the production process of just 1 kg of soybeans (a major component of several animal feeds) produces 7.7 kgs of GHGs. Other contributors include rampant deforestation for livestock maintenance accounting for 9 percent and animal emissions (39 percent) as well as the decomposition of animal waste (10 percent).

Land use – the increasing demand to feed massive populations across the world is putting enormous pressure on our lands. A staggering 75 percent of total agricultural land use is dedicated to livestock production with a significant portion used to grow animal feeds. By cutting down on livestock produce such as beef, poultry, and pork, we can significantly reduce the demand for land use dedicated to livestock production and possible feed more than 4 billion people in addition to our current capacity.

Health – excessive meat consumption is associated with a long list of diseases including cancer, heart problems, stroke, and obesity. According to a research conducted by Friends of the Earth, a low-meat diet could significantly lower premature deaths by 45,000 and save 1.2 billion GBP in medical services. By fully committing to a flexitarian diet, you can save thousands of dollars from hospitalization and medicine while reducing your risk to contract heart diseases, obesity, stroke, and other fatal illnesses.

The livestock industry plays a vital role in the lives of 1 billion of the world's poorest communities. It also provides sources of income for billions worldwide while being the primary source of food of the other billions living in more developed countries. Following a flexitarian diet does not mean abandoning the entire livestock industry and letting the people relying on livestock to suffer and lose their source of income. After all, there is a big difference between big livestock producers compared to small-scale livestock ventures – with the latter being the source of income for the poorest peoples of the world.

Indeed, following a flexitarian diet has a great deal of benefits not just at the individual level, but also to the environment as a whole. In addition to improving your overall health and life expectancy, the flexitarian diet reduces your carbon footprint while also reducing the demand for meat consumption worldwide.

The unsustainable practice of excessive meat consumption has placed a huge toll on the planet. From desertification, acidification, deforestation to higher GHG emissions, the demand for greater meat and processed food production is facilitating greater damage to the environment. With the flexitarian diet as a sustainable dietary alternative, we can begin to turn the tables around and tread a more sustainable path.

Chapter 3: Your Step by Step Guide

Now equipped with the benefits of living a flexitarian lifestyle as well as a general idea of how the flexitarian diet works, there is no reason not to begin your diet today.

Some individuals may find it difficult to transition from being a regular meat eater into a flexitarian. After all, 26 ounces of meat per week is a drastic change in dietary patterns that can mess up your digestive system and your metabolism. The main transitioning problem is the lack of iron and vitamin B complex from most plant-based food. But fret not as there are plenty of plant-based alternatives that are also excellent sources of iron and B vitamins. These meat alternatives will be discussed in succeeding sections.

Before you start, there are things that you need to do first to ensure smooth transition.

Important Things that You Must Do First

1. You need to store more vegetables than meat in your refrigerator and change the way you buy your supply.

It is recommended to buy your ingredients at your local grocery or better yet, plant your own vegetables to make sure that you will always have your supply of organic produce. It is best to use the vegetables in season. Just buy the amount of meat that you need to use in your meal plan for the week to avoid consuming more than the required portion that you intend to eat. When buying meat, make sure to be conscious about not consuming processed food as these types of meat can have a huge toll on your health and may even reverse years of flexitarian re-programming.

2. Gather the flexitarian recipes that you want to collect and make sure to include more variety of vegetable recipes and just enough meat recipes.

Aside from the recipes that this book provides, you can also use your own collection of flexitarian recipes to plan your meal. It may be quite challenging to make a weekly plan at first, but you will soon get the hang of it. You can also bring your own lunch and snacks to the office. As you continue following this book in the following months or years, you will begin to realize that you can invent new dishes and create new recipes based on your experience of eating less meat. We encourage you to nurture these recipes and gather them not just for personal use, but also to share to your friends and family in the aim of providing more meat-free alternatives.

3. Look for vegetable and meat stores that sell organic commodities.

As much as possible, avoid consuming foods that have preservatives or pesticides. Always choose organic if you want keep your body in peak of health. Choose free range meat and organic produce. If it's inevitable to avoid canned goods and processed meats, then make sure to consume them in moderation.

4. Start eating more vegetables and other fares in the additional food groups.

Before you plan your flexitarian meal, you can start consuming more vegetables than your usual intake. You also need to increase your meat alternatives. Try to cut your meat consumption, but don't force yourself. Take it as a trial phase as you introduce your taste buds to the different flavors of vegetables. Your body might have to adjust due to the fact that eating 26 ounces of meet per week is a drastic dietary change that can make your metabolism go haywire. But don't worry because there are a lot of things you can do to stop this from happening. Start consuming more vegetables in a gradual pacing and work your way into transitioning to more-veggie, less-meat diets.

Time to Start

Once you have everything that you need and your body has begun adjusting to a semi-vegetarian diet, it is time to start. It is important that you have familiarized yourself with the different food groups and began eating more vegetables than meat. You are about to reduce your meat consumption further from this point onwards.

1. There's no need for you to rush everything, what you need is to make sure that you can commit yourself to the diet. You can start with meat-free Monday, where you commit yourself not to include meat in your diet for a single day in a week. As you proceed with following the flexitarian diet, you can continue adding more meatless days in your week until you reach a once a month meatless day.
2. Consume more greens by whipping up a fulfilling garden salad. You can try different salad dressings on your choice of greens. You can even use the same combinations of green, leafy vegetables and toss them in different salad dressings each day or each meal. The dressing can help create a different taste to the usual greens.

You can start with these greens for your salad: 3 to 4 cups lettuce of any variety, kale, arugula, or kale together with carrots, beets, onion, or broccoli. You can experiment with other greens as well.

3. Stock up on spices. The inventive meatless choices that a flexitarian lifestyle offers you are basically endless. To make your culinary experience more delectable, it is best to stock up on your spice selections. You can begin with paprika and other chili and pepper variations to add spice to your garden salads and tomato-based food. Start investing in basil, mint, sage, cloves, and work your way to introducing more and more spices to your taste palette. It is also worth noting that spices are also important in stimulating your metabolism which is a good thing when you're on a flexitarian diet.

4. Look up the recipes that this book provides and plan your meal for a week. You can also include the recipes that you have collected. You will improve your meal planning as time goes on. You also need to remember to consume smaller portions of meat so you get used to the diet in a matter of time.
4. Don't forget to drink lots of water and add physical activities in your daily routine. Water intake is a crucial element in any diet – whether flexitarian or any other diet. Make sure to drink at least 8 glasses a day. You may need to add more based on the physical activities and sweat you produce as waste every single day.
5. If you are a smoker, it is best to cut down the number of cigarettes that you puff in a day. It is best if you can eliminate it completely. You need to drink alcohol in moderation. Alcohol moderation is crucial in keeping up with your caloric requirements. Drinking alcohol more than a few times a week or month can lead you to gain more calories than you think you are getting from a flexitarian diet. You can refer to this **link** to know the calorie content of your favorite drink. (http://www.the-alcoholism-guide.org/alcohol-calorie-chart.html)
6. Stick to the routine and you will soon reap the benefits that you want to gain. No pain, no gain right? In this case, there's really no pain involved. But what the flexitarian diet entails is a serious amount of dedication and determination. While it does not demand the same amount of effort demanded by purely vegetarian diets, it does not mean that flexitarianism is just a walk in the park. Commit to the flexitarian diet and you will soon reap the benefits of a flexitarian lifestyle.

High-Protein Vegetarian Alternatives

Now, you might be wondering if meat is such an essential part of the human body's regular dietary requirements, why reduce it to such an amount as 26 ounces per week?

Meat remains the most excellent supplier of dietary protein as well as nutrients such as zinc, iron, and vitamins B1, B2, B3 and B12. Reducing meat intake can actually lead to iron deficiency anemia especially for those who are predisposed to the illness. And while meat is still the most preferred source of protein and micronutrients, it doesn't mean that there is no vegetarian alternative out there.

In fact, you have hundreds of vegan protein meals to choose from – from potatoes, green peas, beans, quinoa, tofu, and other high-protein crops and vegetables – you'll never run out of protein, iron and essential nutrients again.

To help you in your meal plans, here are a few of the best sources of vegan protein for you to consider:

Source of Vegan Protein	Protein Content (per 100g or 3.5 oz in weight)
Potato	2.50
Brown Rice	2.58
Spinach	2.90
Quinoa	4.40
Kidney Beans	4.83
Pinto Beans	4.86
Green Peas	5.36
Macadamia Nuts	7.79
Lima Beans	7.80
Wheat Bread	8.80
Garbanzo Beans	8.90
Lentils	9.02
Pecans	9.50
Soybeans	13.10
Walnuts	15.03

Hazelnuts	15.03
Cashew Nuts	15.31
Chia Seeds	15.60
Oats	16.89
Tofu	17.19
Flaxseed	19.50
Pistachio Nuts	21.35
Almonds	22.09
Hemp Seed	23.00
Peanut Butter	25.09
Pumpkin Seeds	32.97

Some Important Tips

1. Try eating legumes, such as lentils, chickpeas, and white beans. You can have nuts for your snack.
2. Instead of eating chicken, beef, or pork, try substituting it with a cup of beans or lentils. It is definitely filling, although not as tasty as meat. But lentils and beans can also provide the same amount of protein that meat has.
3. You can also substitute your meat with tofu, tempeh, and other soy-based fares. Soy-based food is also a good substitute for meat especially for beginner flexitarians who are starting to miss the texture of meaty dishes. Try a delicious tofu recipe and re-live the glory of pork cutlets melting in your mouth!
4. Focus on foods that have low calories and abundant in nutrients. As you progress, you need to add more vegetables and other protein sources apart from meat.
5. You can also have quinoa in your diet. It is an amazing grain that contains adequate amount of protein.

Don’t forget to eat the mentioned foods along with your whole grains, greens, and/or fruits.

You can also refer to this table when planning your meal:

CALORIES	SIZE	FOOD
2	regular	Coffee (black, brewed)
6	2 tsps	Yellow mustard
15	1 tbsp	Ketchup
35	4 ounces	Salsa
40	1 cup	Canned green beans
52	1 cup	Raw carrots
59	1 small piece	Chocolate chip cookie
59	plain	Graham cracker (cinnamon, plain, or honey)
66	1 slice	Bread (white or wheat)
72	1 medium	Apple
84	3 ounces	Cooked shrimp (cooked under moist heat)
92	4 ounces	Spaghetti sauce (ready to serve, marinara)
100	3 ounces	Canned tuna in water (light)
102	large	Egg (scrambled)
102	1 tbsp	Salted butter
105	1 medium	Banana
108	1 ounce	Pretzels (crunchy, salted, plain)
112	8 ounces	Frozen concentrate orange juice
113	1 slice	Cheddar cheese
121	5 ounces	White wine
122	8 ounces	Milk (2% fat)
123	5 ounces	Red wine
130	1.5 ounces	Raisins
136	12 ounces	Cola
137	1 piece	Hot dog (pork and beef)

142	3 ounces	Chicken breast (roasted, skinless, boneless)
145	4 ounces	Vanilla ice cream
146	2 tbsps	Salad dressing (ranch)
147	1 cup	Oatmeal (regular, cooked in plain water)
155	1 ounce	Salted potato chips (plain)
161	medium	Potato (baked, skin intact)
168	1 ounce	Dry roasted mixed nuts (salted with peanuts)
180	2 tbsps	Creamy peanut butter
180	1 cup	Whole kernel sweet yellow corn
193	4 ounces	Beef patty (ground, 15% fat, pan-broiled):
193	1.5-ounce	Granola raisin bar
205	1 cup	Cooked rice (long grain, white)
221	3 ounces	Broiled Pork chop (boneless)
221	1 cup	Spaghetti (cooked)
243	1 piece	Yellow cake with chocolate frosting
287	1 cup	Canned chili with beans
289	1 medium	Bagel
289	1 piece	Jelly doughnut
298	1 slice	Regular crust pepperoni pizza

Chapter 4: Breakfast Recipes

Breakfast is the most important meal of the day. Some diet techniques actually recommend doing away with breakfast altogether, but the Flexitarian diet celebrates this nutritious habit with a flexitarian twist. This chapter contains the recipes that you can try for breakfast. The breakfast recipes included in this chapter are meant to give you that extra boost you need to start the day while fulfilling the caloric intake requirements as set out in earlier chapters.

Oat and Blueberry Pancakes with Yogurt

Prep Time : 10 minutes

Cook Time : 36 minutes

Total Calories : 400

Servings : 2

You will need:

2 large eggs, beaten
1 cup blueberries
1 tbsp maple syrup
1/2 cup low-fat cottage cheese
3/4 cup plain low-fat Greek yogurt
1 teaspoon vanilla extract
1 cup old-fashioned rolled oats
Cooking spray

Procedure:

1. Combine eggs, cottage cheese, vanilla, and oats in a blender and process until you obtain a smooth consistency.
2. Add the blueberries and stir them in (don't pulse the blender). Divide the mixture into 6 equal portions.
3. Put a large nonstick pan over medium heat. Coat it with cooking spray.
4. Pour a portion of the batter and cook for 3 minutes. Flip it and cook the other side for another 3 minutes.
5. Get a small bowl and combine maple syrup and yogurt. Mix well. Divide the mixture into two equal parts.
6. Each pancake serving comes with yogurt-maple syrup mixture.

Maple and Vanilla French Toast with Saucy Raspberry

Prep Time	: 10 minutes
Cook Time	: 12 minutes
Total Calories	: 300
Servings	: 2

You will need:

2 slices bread, whole-grain
1 whole egg
2 egg whites
1/4 cup raspberries
1 tsp maple syrup
1/4 tsp vanilla extract
1 tsp fresh lemon juice
Cooking spray

Procedure:

1. Put the egg, egg whites, vanilla, and maple syrup in a bowl and whisk.
2. Coat a nonstick pan with cooking spray and put over medium heat.
3. Dip each slice of bread in the egg mixture and cook each side for 3 minutes.
4. Mash raspberries in a bowl and add lemon juice. Blend well. Pour the mixture over the toasts.

Asian Fusion Mushroom Pastry (Family Meal for 6pax)

Prep Time	: 55 minutes
Cook Time	: 10-15 minutes (oven included)
Total Calories	: 327
Servings	: 6

You will need:

100g chestnut mushrooms (8.8 oz)
2 tbsp coriander
35g carrots
½ tsp Chinese 5 Spice Mix
2 diced shallots
1 tsp soy sauce
1 sliced and crushed garlic clove
1 tbsp breadcrumbs
1 chia egg (1 tbsp of ground chia seeds mixed in 1 Tbsp water)
½ puff of pastry sheet
Olive oil
Unsalted butter
Salt
White Pepper

Procedure:

1. Mix the ground chia seeds with water and set aside for a few minutes.

2. Slice the mushrooms into bite-sized pieces or in fine strips depending on your preference.
3. Heat a large skillet and pour the olive oil. Once the skillet is hot enough, add the shallots, garlic, and Chinese 5 Spice mix.
4. Grate the carrots and mix with the minced mushrooms. Fry the carrot-mushroom mix on low-medium heat until mushrooms are cooked and carrots are tender.
5. Set aside the skillet and add the soy sauce, coriander, chia egg mix and breadcrumbs. Mix everything until fully blended and season with salt and pepper.

6. Before preparing the pastry sheets, pre-heat the oven up to 200 degrees Celsius.
7. Carefully place the pastry sheet onto another sheet of baking paper and pour the mixture depending on how much you want each roll to contain.
8. Roll up the pastry sheet onto the mixture and brush with butter.
9. Cook in oven for 24 minutes until the pastry becomes golden brown.
10. Leave the pastry to cool down for at least ten minutes before serving.

Vegetarian Casserole
(Good for 2pax)

Prep Time	: 3 minutes
Cook Time	: 5 minutes (toasting included)
Total Calories	: 300
Servings	: 6

You will need:

1 medium-sized sweet potato
½ small cauliflower head
½ tsp cumin seeds
1 small onion
1 red bell pepper
1 tbsp olive oil (you can use extra virgin olive oil as well)
1 ¼ cups of red salsa
5 corn tortillas
½ can black beans
¼ cup chopped cilantro
1 handful of spinach leaves
½ cup of Shredded Monterey Jack

Procedure:

1. Oven-roast vegetables at 400 degrees Farenheit. Place the vegetables on a baking sheet to avoid sticking.
2. Mix cauliflower head together with cut sweet potato and olive oil in a pan. Heat another pan and mix bell pepper, onion, and olive oil on it. Add cumin seeds on both pans.

3. Drizzle salt and pepper to taste in both pans. Ensure that the mixture becomes coated in spices. Add olive oil whenever you think it is necessary. Oven-bake until vegetables are tender and caramelized.
4. Mix the cilantro with the red salsa. Lower oven temperature to 350 degrees Fahrenheit.
5. Pour in the salsa onto the bottom of the pan. Place a layer of tortilla and make sure it is covered with salsa.
6. Add in the beans, vegetables, spinach and cheese.

7. Carefully create another tortilla layer and pour in all of the remaining salsa, vegetables and Monterey Jack.
8. Repeat the process and cover the pan with parchment paper. Bake for 20 minutes and remove the cover. After a few minutes of cooling down, return the pan back into the oven and heat for another 10 minutes.
9. Remove the pan from the oven and let the casserole cool and dry before serving.

Berry Waffles

Prep Time	: 3 minutes
Cook Time	: 5 minutes (toasting included)
Total Calories	: 300
Servings	: 2

You will need:

1 tbsp maple syrup
1/2 frozen mixed berries, thawed
2 whole-grain waffles (frozen)

Procedure:

1. Toast the waffles.
2. Put the berries in a microwavable bowl and mash them. Add in syrup and mix well.
3. Microwave for 30 seconds and pour the mixture on toasted waffles.

Zucchini, Feta, and Mint Fritters

Prep Time : 10 minutes
Cook Time : 10 minutes
Total Calories : 80
Servings : 5

You will need:

50 g feta, cubed
Handful of fresh mint, torn
2 eggs
5 pieces medium zucchini, grated
Coconut oil for frying

Procedure:

1. Squeeze out the water from the grated zucchini and place it in a large bowl.
2. Add the rest of the ingredients and combine well.
3. Divide the mixture into ten equal portions.
4. Put the frying pan over medium heat. Make sure that the pan is hot enough before adding the coconut oil.
5. Fry the fritters until golden brown. You may need to cook them in batches.

Chapter 5: Veggie galore (lunch and dinner)

Vegan recipes are not everyone's cup of tea. But with a little twist, those old veggie dishes that you used to hate when you were a kid will become heaven to your adult taste buds. Try these succulent veggie recipes...with a twist!

Mushroom Quinoa Delight

Prep Time : 15 minutes

Cook Time : 30 minutes

Total Calories : 211.9 per serving

Serving : 5

You will need:

Burger Recipe:

4 Chopped medium mushrooms (without gills)
¼ cup chopped red onion
1 cup quinoa
3 chopped green onions
½ cup of cornstarch
1 garlic clove
Buns
Sliced Tomatoes
Sprouts

Dressing Recipe:

1 tsp rosemary
½ cup of mayonnaise
Salt and pepper to taste
1 tsp lemon juice

Procedure:

1. To make the burgers, you first have to preheat the oven to 375 degrees Farenheit. In a shallow baking dish, place the mushrooms with garlic, 1 tablespoon of oil, ¾ teaspoon salt, and ¼ teaspoon pepper. Spread it evenly across the baking dish. Bake for 20 minutes or until mushrooms are tender. Set aside to cool and turn off oven.

2. Place the mushroom mixture together with red onion, green onions, and vinegar until mixture becomes homogenous. Transfer the paste to a large bowl and stir together with quinoa and cornstarch until everything is well-blended. Cover the bowl with cling wrap and put in a refrigerator for 2 hours.

3. Preheat the oven to 375 degrees F. Place a baking sheet with foil. Create burger patties from the mixture (makes up to 5 patties of 1/2 inch thickness and 3 inches wide.

4. In a medium skillet, heat oil and pan-sear the burger patties until browned. Place the pan-seared patties back to the baking sheet and bake for 10 minutes in the oven.

5. To make the dressing, combine the mayonnaise, rosemary, lemon juice and a pinch of salt.

6. Serve burgers on buns with Rosemary Mayo dressing. Garnish with sprouts, lettuce and tomatoes.

Feta-Spinach Pie

Prep Time : 25 minutes
Cook Time : 50 minutes
Total Calories : 209
Servings : 10

For the pie crust, you will need:

1 egg
150 g almond flour
Salt and pepper
1 tbsp coconut flour

Procedure for the pie:

1. Combine all ingredients in a bowl and mix them thoroughly using a fork.
2. Get a 24cm x 9.5 inch pie tin and lightly grease the entire surface.
3. Pour the pie mixture in the pie tin. Get a clean drinking glass and use its base to smooth out the pie crust. Make sure to fill the pie tin evenly. You may need to use a piece of baking paper on the surface of the crust before you smooth it out.
4. Prick the base of the crust using fork.
5. Bake the pie crust at 350°F for 15 minutes. Set aside.

For the pie filling, you will need:

6 eggs, lightly beaten
150 g feta, crumbled
500 g fresh spinach
1/2 onion, finely chopped
Handful of fresh mint, torn
Salt and pepper
250 g cream cheese (use full fat)

Procedure for the filling:

1. Make sure to squeeze out the water from your spinach when you wash it – you don't want a soggy pie.
2. Combine the spinach and the rest of the ingredients in a large bowl.
3. Mix gently and make sure to leave some feta and cream cheese lumps.
4. Pour mixture onto the prepared pie crust.

5. Bake at 350°F for 35 minutes or until the center is cooked.

Green Fatty Pizza

Prep Time	: 10 minutes
Cook Time	: 25 minutes
Total Calories	: 203
Servings	: 6

For pizza base, you will need:

1 whole egg
1/2 tsp dried rosemary
2 tbsps cream cheese
85 g almond meal
170 g mozzarella, shredded
100 g fresh spinach, chopped
Salt and pepper to taste

For pizza toppings, you will need:

1 medium zucchini, finely sliced
Feta, crumbled
1/8 cup spring onion, coarsely chopped
1/4 cup fresh mint, coarsely chopped

Procedure:

1. Get a microwavable bowl. Put almond flour and mozzarella in it and combine well. Put the cream cheese in. Set the microwave to high and melt the cheese for one minute.
2. Stir the mixture and microwave for another 25 seconds.
3. Add salt, egg, and rosemary. Combine everything carefully.
4. Get two pieces of parchment paper and put the pizza base in between them. Roll it out with a rolling pin and try to make a circular shape. Peel off the parchment paper on top.
5. Get a fork and make several tiny holes on the pizza base.
6. Put the pizza base (bottom parchment paper still intact) on a baking tray and bake at 425°F for 10 to 16 minutes.
7. Remove the pizza base from the oven and start spreading the toppings on top. Finish off with crumbled feta.

8. Pop it in the oven once more using the same temperature and bake for 6 to 7 minutes.

Asian Zucchini Salad

Prep Time	: 10 minutes
Cook Time	: n/a
Total Calories	: 120
Servings	: 2

You will need:

1 medium zucchini, sliced thinly into spirals
1/3 cup rice vinegar
3/4 cup avocado oil
1 cup sunflower seeds, shells removed
1 lb cabbage, shredded
1 tsp stevia drops
1 cup almonds, sliced

Procedure:

1. Cut the zucchini spirals into smaller parts. Set aside.
2. Put almonds, sunflower seeds, and cabbage in a large bowl. Combine the ingredients well.
3. Add zucchini in the mixture.
4. Get a small bowl and mix vinegar, stevia, and oil using a whisk or fork.
5. Pour the vinegar mixture all over the zucchini mixture. Toss well and make sure that everything is covered with the dressing.
6. Refrigerate for 2 hours before serving.

Mushroom and Spinach Pie with no Crust

Prep Time : 15 minutes
Cook Time : 60 minutes
Total Calories : 266
Servings : 6

You will need:

16 ounces 4% cottage cheese
4 eggs
10 ounces fresh spinach
8 ounces fresh mushrooms, sliced thinly
1/2 mozzarella, shredded
1/4 tsp nutmeg
2 tsps oil
1/2 cup heavy cream
1 tsp minced garlic
1/2 tsp pepper
2 tbsps parmesan, grated
1 tsp salt

Procedure:

1. Preheat oven to 350°F.
2. Put a large skillet over medium heat. When the surface is hot enough, add oil. Sauté garlic and add mushrooms. Cook until tender.
3. Add spinach, nutmeg, pepper, and salt. Stir for a bit and cook until spinach is cooked.
4. Pour the cooked spinach mixture in a colander to drain.
5. Get a 9-inch pie dish and sprinkle it with parmesan until the entire surface is covered with cheese.
6. Get a bowl and whisk the eggs. Add cottage cheese and cream to the egg and mix well.
7. Add in the spinach and mushroom mixture.
8. Transfer the spinach mixture onto the pie dish. Top with more mozzarella.
9. Arrange the pie dish on a baking tray and bake for 50 to 60 minutes.
10. Turn off the oven and let the pie sit for 10 minutes before taking it out.

11. Let it rest at room temperature for 10 minutes before slicing.

Mini Eggplant Parmesan

Prep Time	: 15 minutes
Cook Time	: 20 minutes
Total Calories	: 72
Servings	: 10

You will need:

1 large eggplant, sliced into 10 equal parts
1 egg, beaten
Salt and pepper to taste
25 g parmesan, shredded
50 g cheddar cheese, grated
1 tsp thyme
1 tsp rosemary
25 g almond flour

Procedure:

1. Grease a baking dish and arrange the eggplant slices on top. Sprinkle with salt and pepper.
2. Bake at 350°F until golden brown.
3. While waiting for the eggplant to cook, get a medium bowl and combine the herbs, cheeses, and flour together. Mix well. Divide the mixture into 10 equal parts.
4. Remove the eggplant from the oven when done. Turn each slice over and season with salt and pepper. Pop it to the oven once more and cook until golden brown.
5. Remove the cooked eggplant from the oven and brush beaten egg on top of each eggplant slice.
6. Put a portion of herb and cheese mixture on each slice. Put the eggplant back into the oven and bake until the cheese begins to melt.

Chapter 6: Guilt-Free Meat and Meat Alternatives (Lunch and Dinner)

The main selling point of a flexitarian diet is you get to live the best of both worlds. Eating your favorite meaty dishes combined with the most inventive vegan delights has never been this fun (and nutritious!).
Here are some meat dishes for you to enjoy (in regulation).

Horseradish Aioli and Roast Beef Sandwich

Prep Time	: 10 minutes
Cook Time	: n/a
Total Calories	: 359
Serving	: 1

You will need:
1 tbsp low-fat, less sodium Italian dressing
2 ounces roast beef, sliced
2 tbsps reduced-fat mayonnaise
1 small cucumber, sliced
2 slices rye bread
1/2 cup fresh spinach
2 tsps prepared horseradish
Procedure:
1. In a small bowl, combine horseradish and mayonnaise and stir well.
2. Put some mayonnaise mixture on each slice of bread.
3. Arrange the roast beef slices and spinach on one slice of bread and top it with the other slice of bread.
4. Serve the sandwich with slices of cucumber with dressing.

Yummy BLT

Prep Time	: 6 minutes
Cook Time	: 2 minutes

Total Calories : 400

Servings : 2

You will need:

1 tbsp light mayonnaise

4 slices turkey bacon

2 slices whole-grain bread

2 leaves romaine lettuce

2 tomato slices

Procedure:

1. Toast the 2 slices of bread and microwave bacon for 2 to 3 minutes.
2. Spread some mayonnaise on one side of a slice of bread.
3. Add bacon, lettuce, and tomato on the side of bread with mayonnaise. Cover it with the other slice of bread.
4. Cut diagonally and serve.

Tuna and Veggies Wrap

Prep Time : 10 minutes

Cook Time : n/a

Total Calories : 400

Servings : 2

You will need:

2 pieces whole-grain tortillas
1 cup cucumber, sliced
1 tbsp low-fat Italian dressing
1 cup carrots, julienned

Procedure:

1. Put the dressing and tuna in a bowl and mix well.
2. Arrange half of the mixture on one of the tortillas. Add half the amount of each vegetable and wrap.
3. Do the same to the remaining tortilla.

Strips of Chicken Barbeque Wrap

Prep Time : 10 minutes
Cook Time : n/a
Total Calories : 400
Servings : 2

You will need:

5 ounces left-over or pre-cooked chicken, cut in strips
2 tbsps barbecue sauce
1 large whole-grain tortilla
1/4 cup broccoli, shredded and blanched
1/4 cup carrot, shredded and blanched
1/4 cup cauliflower, shredded and blanched
1/4 cup cabbage, shredded and blanched

Procedure:

1. Put all the shredded vegetables in a bowl and toss to combine well.
2. Spread the tortilla. Put the barbecue sauce, strips of chicken, and mixed veggies.
3. Wrap everything, cut in half (secure each half with a toothpick), and serve.

Chestnut and Mushroom Rolls

Prep Time : 25 minutes

Cook Time : 25 minutes

Total Calories : 211.9

Servings : 20 bite-sized squares

You will need:

100g chestnut mushrooms
Puff pastry sheets
1 clove garlic
1 dried thyme
250g of mushroom
200g breadcrumbs
1 tsp black pepper
1 tsp salt
1 tbsp poppy seeds
1 tbsp vegan spread

Procedure:

1. First, preheat the oven up to a temperature of 180 degrees Celsius.
2. Drizzle olive oil onto a large skillet and cook in medium heat. Throw in diced onion and cook for another 10 minutes until onions are translucent.
3. Mix garlic and thyme and stir for another minute before pouring in the mushrooms. Stir-fry the mushrooms until it becomes limp and golden brown.
4. Drain excessive liquid from the pan. Once drained, mix in the chestnuts.
5. Add some sherry and cook for another 5 minutes before plating it for serving.
6. Carefully place the mixture onto the rolled out pastry puff.
7. Add the breadcrumbs, pepper, salt and sage. Mix until well-blended. Form a crumbly ball with the mixture and split the ball into four equal sizes. One ball of mixture goes into each strip of puff pastry.

8. Form a sausage-shaped pastry roll. Brush the whole pastry with vegan spread and cut it into 2-cm bite-sized pieces. Place in a baking pan with baking sheet lining. Sprinkle some poppy seeds and oven cook for 20-25 minutes until golden brown.
10. Let the mixture cool before serving

Guilt-Free Egg Salad

Prep Time	: 10 minutes
Cook Time	: 5 minutes
Total Calories	: 205
Servings	: 4

You will need:

125 ml mayonnaise (choose full fat variety)
6 eggs, hard boiled
Some fresh parsley, chopped
1 tsp. curry powder or to taste

Procedure:

1. Peel the cooked eggs and chop them coarsely. Put the chopped eggs in a large bowl.
2. Add mayonnaise and curry powder into the bowl and blend well.
3. Sprinkle with parsley and serve.

Chapter 7: Easy Snacks and Drinks

Quick and easy snack recipes are a must if you're the type of person who craves for bite-sized munchies in between regular meals. Especially on a flexitarian diet, snacks and drinks are an important part of the day. In addition to quenching your thirst, in-between meals give you the extra boost of energy you need to get through the day.
These snacks and drinks are simple and easy to prepare, check them out.

Veggies and Cottage Cheese Dip

Prep Time	: 10 minutes
Cook Time	: n/a
Total Calories	: 120
Serving	: 1

You will need:
1/2 cup baby carrots, blanched
1/2 cup snow peas, blanched
1/4 tsp lemon pepper
1/2 cup cottage cheese (choose low-fat)

Procedure:
1. Put all cottage cheese and lemon pepper in a bowl. Mix well.
2. Arrange the baby carrots, peas, and dip in a platter. Serve.

You can also replace the carrots and peas with different vegetables.

Toast with Baked Beans

Prep Time	: 15 minutes
Cook Time	: 10 minutes
Total Calories	: 83
Serving	: 2

You will need:

½ tbsp olive oil (preferably extra virgin)
1 tbsp ketchup
¼ tsp apple cider vinegar
¼ tsp mustard powder
Pepper
½ tsp Worcestershire sauce
1 tbsp + 1tsp maple syrup
1 tsp molasses
1 can of drained and rinsed navy beens

Procedure:

1. Saute onion with olive oil in a medium skillet. Cook until onions are limp.
2. Mix all of the remaining ingredients and stir well over low-medium heat for about 5-10 minutes until all ingredients are cooked. Add salt and pepper to taste.
3. Let the dish cool for 5 minutes before serving with fresh toast.

Raspberry Sauce on Watermelon

Prep Time : 15 minutes

Cook Time : n/a

Total Calories : 83

Serving : 1

You will need:

3 pieces kiwi fruit, peeled and sliced
2 tbsps sugar
3 tbsps orange juice
1 small cantaloupe, cut in half and seeds removed
1 pint strawberries, cut in half
1pint blueberries
1/2 seedless watermelon, rind removed and cut in bite size
1 1/2 cups frozen raspberries, thawed

Procedure:

1. Get a melon baller and scoop out the cantaloupe flesh.
2. Put the watermelon pieces in the center of a plate. Arrange the remaining fruits around the watermelon.
3. Get a blender put in orange juice, raspberries, and sugar. Process everything until smooth.
4. Pour the mixture over the fruits in the plate.

No-Dairy Strawberry Smoothie

Prep Time : 5 minutes
Cook Time : n/a
Total Calories : 152
Servings : 2 glasses

You will need:
2 cups of fresh strawberries
1 banana
2 tbsps maple syrup
¼ cup non-dairy milk

Procedure:
Mix together all of the ingredients into a food processor or blender.
Pour onto two glasses and enjoy.

Green Chocolate Smoothie

Prep Time : 10 minutes

Cook Time : n/a

Total Calories : 186

Servings : 2

You will need:

250 ml coconut cream
25 g cocoa powder
50 g of your favorite berries, frozen
100 g fresh spinach, chopped
1 tbsp. granulated sugar or to taste

Procedure:

1. Put all the ingredients in a blender and process until smooth. Make it as smooth as possible.
2. Pour in a tall glass and enjoy.

Peach and Raspberry Smoothie

Prep Time : 7 minutes
Cook Time : n/a
Total Calories : 65
Servings : 2

You will need:

3/4 cup apple juice
1 cup peaches, frozen
1 cup raspberries, frozen
6 ounces non-fat yogurt (plain)

Procedure:

1. Drop all the ingredients in a blender and pulse until smooth.
2. Pour in a tall glass and enjoy.

Chapter 8: 5-Day Meal Plan

Now that you're almost ready to get started, the first thing you have to do is to formulate your own plan based on all of the information provided in previous chapters and your knowledge of protein-calorie content of certain foods. To help you get started, here is a sample 5-day meal plan:

	Day 1	Day 2	Day 3	Day 4	Day 5
Breakfast	Oat and Blueberry Pancakes with Yogurt, apple(medium)	1 slice bread (wheat or white), 1 tbsp salted butter, 1 piece hotdog	Maple and Vanilla French Toast with Saucy Raspberry, 3 ounces chicken breast (roasted, skinless, boneless)	2 servings of Berry Waffles	Oat and Blueberry Pancakes with Yogurt
Snack	Peach and Raspberry Smoothie, 1 ounce pretzels (crunchy, salted, plain)	Veggies and Cottage Cheese Dip	Green Chocolate Smoothie, 2 pieces Chocolate chip cookie (small)	8 ounces milk (2% fat), 1 piece chocolate chip cookie (small)	Raspberry Sauce on Watermelon, 1 slice bread
Lunch	Horseradish Aioli and Roast Beef Sandwich, 1 cup green beans	2 servings of Tuna and Veggies Wrap	2 servings of Mushroom and Spinach Pie with no Crust, 1 cup chili with beans	2 servings of Strips of Chicken Barbeque Wrap	1 medium bagel , 1 slice cheddar cheese
Snack	Green Chocolate Smoothie	Raspberry Sauce on Watermelon	Peach and Raspberry Smoothie	2 pieces chocolate chip cookie (small)	Ice cream (vanilla)
Dinner	2 servings of Strips of Chicken Barbeque Wrap, Guilt-Free Egg Salad	Horseradish Aioli and Roast Beef Sandwich, Asian Zucchini Salad, Peach Raspberry Smoothie	2 servings of Tuna and Veggies Wrap, Green Chocolate Smoothie	6 servings of Mushroom and Spinach Pie with no Crust, 1 medium banana, 8 ounces orange juice	1 whole Feta-Spinach Pie, 1 serving Asian Zucchini Salad, 1 serving Yummy BLT, black coffee

The 5-day meal plan above is just a recommendation. You can change any part of the meal as you go on, but make sure to follow the beginner phase (26 ounces of meat per week) requirements. Also, make it a point to study the calorie counting method and protein content table mentioned in previous chapters.

Conclusion

Thank you again for downloading this book!

I hope this book was able to help you plan and prepare your flexitarian meal that even your whole family can enjoy.

It is not difficult to follow a flexitarian diet, but you still need patience and discipline to succeed. But the important point about the flexitarian diet is that it does not place too much restriction on the way we eat. Instead, it provides alternatives and even celebrates nutritious food (including meat). The only major adjustment you have to make if you are to take this journey is to cut down on meat consumption which, based on previous chapters, is actually a good thing. In addition to shedding off some calories, you can also make a contribution toward preserving the environment while you're at it.

It is important to continue eating flexitarian breakfast, lunch, dinner, and snacks all the time. Do remember that it's best to abstain from eating fast food or store-bought packed lunch as well as other food products that are loaded with preservatives.

If you will continue to follow the flexitarian diet, you will soon feel better than ever before and you will practically shine with youthful glow.

If you enjoyed this book, please take the time to share your thoughts and post a review on Amazon. It'd be greatly appreciated!

Thank you and good luck!

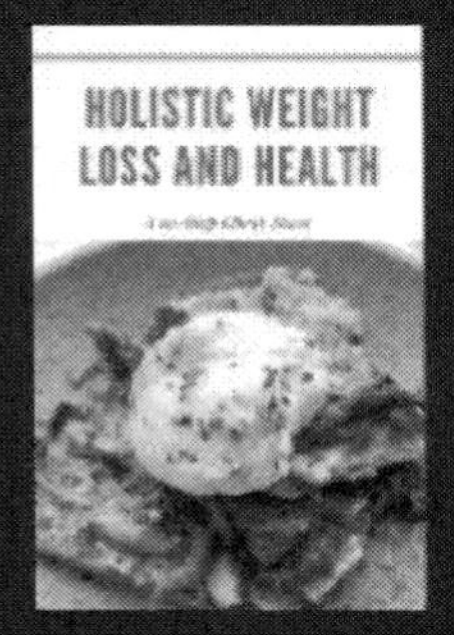
HOLISTIC WEIGHT
LOSS AND HEALTH

Made in the USA
Middletown, DE
21 March 2021